Understanding cancer of the lung

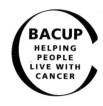

BACUP
HELPING
PEOPLE
LIVE WITH
CANCER

This booklet is for you if you have or someone close to you has cancer of the lung. It has been prepared and checked by cancer doctors, other relevant specialists, nurses and patients. Together they represent an agreed view on this cancer, its diagnosis and management, and the key aspects of living with it.

If you are a patient, your doctor or nurse may wish to go through the booklet with you and mark sections that are particularly important for you. You can make a note below of the main contacts and information that you may need quickly.

Specialist nurse/contact name	Family doctor
. . . .	. . . .
. . . .	. . . .

Hospi   y address

GW00631128

Phone . . . .   If you like, you can also add:

Treatments . . . .   **Your name** . . . .

. . . .   **Address**. . . . .

. . . .

This booklet aims to tell you about cancer of the lung, how it is diagnosed and treated and how the treatment may affect you.

These two pages sum up the main points, and show which pages to turn to for more information.

What causes cancer of the lung? Page 9

- smoking is the cause of the great majority of lung cancers

- inhaling other people's cigarette smoke **(passive smoking)** slightly increases the risk of developing lung cancer

- high levels of a naturally occurring gas called **radon gas** may also increase the risk of developing lung cancer

- exposure to some substances such as asbestos, uranium, chromium and nickel has been linked to lung cancer but these are very rare causes

What are the symptoms of cancer of the lung? Page 10

The symptoms may include any of the following:

- a persistent cough or change in the nature of a long-standing cough

- a chest infection that does not get better

- shortness of breath

- coughing up blood-stained phlegm

- chest discomfort (a dull ache or a sharp pain when you cough or take a deep breath)

- loss of appetite and weight

One or more of the following tests may be used:

- chest X-ray
- sputum cytology
- bronchoscopy
- mediastinoscopy
- lung biopsy

- CT scan
- liver and upper abdominal ultrasound scan
- isotope bone scan

Surgery, radiotherapy and chemotherapy may be used, alone or together, to treat cancer of the lung.

You may feel anxious, afraid or angry because of the cancer, the treatment and its effects.

The worst fear is often fear of the unknown.

It may help you to find out as much as you can about the cancer, its treatment, and living with it.

Do not be afraid to ask, and go on asking until you get the information and support you need.

For more information

Many people and organisations can help. This booklet lists useful organisations (page 37), books that might help (page 40), and BACUP's booklets (page 42).

The nurses in BACUP's cancer information service (0171 613 2121 or Freephone 0800 18 11 99) can give information about all aspects of cancer, and people who can help.

If you need to talk through your feelings in depth, you can contact BACUP's cancer counselling service on 0171 696 9000, or at BACUP Scotland in Glasgow on 0141 553 1553.

3 Bath Place, Rivington Street, London, EC2A 3JR

BACUP was founded by Dr Vicky Clement-Jones, following her own experiences with ovarian cancer, and offers information, counselling and support to people with cancer, their families and friends.

We produce publications on the main types of cancer, treatments, and ways of living with cancer. We also produce a magazine, *BACUP News,* three times a year.

Our success depends on feedback from users of the service. We thank everyone, particularly patients and their families, whose advice has made this booklet possible.

Administration 0171 696 9003
Cancer Support Service:
Information 0171 613 2121 (8 lines) or Freeline 0800 18 11 99
Counselling 0171 696 9000 (London)
BACUP Scotland Cancer Counselling Service
0141 553 1553 (Glasgow)

British Association of Cancer United Patients and their families and friends.
A company limited by guarantee. Registered in England and Wales
company number 2803321. Charity registration number 1019719.
Registered office 3 Bath Place, Rivington Street, London, EC2A 3JR

Medical consultant: Dr Maurice Slevin, MD, FRCP

Editor: Stella Wood

Text illustration: Andrew Macdonald

Cover design: Alison Hooper Associates

First published 1987, revised editions 1990, 1994, 1996, 1997
© BACUP 1987, 1990, 1994, 1995, 1996, 1997

Typeset and printed in Great Britain by Lithoflow Ltd., London

ISBN 1-901276-02-3

Contents

Introduction

This information booklet has been written to help you understand more about cancer of the lung. We hope it answers some of the questions you may have about its diagnosis and treatment, and addresses some of the feelings which are a large part of anyone's reaction to a cancer diagnosis.

We can't advise you about the best treatment for yourself because this information can only come from your own doctor, who will be familiar with your full medical history.

At the end of this booklet you will find a list of other BACUP publications, some useful addresses and recommended books, and a page to fill in with any questions you may have for your doctor or nurse. If, after reading this booklet, you think it has helped you, do pass it on to any of your family and friends who might find it interesting. They too may want to be informed so they can help you cope with any problems you may have.

What is cancer?

The organs and tissues of the body are made up of tiny building blocks called cells. Cancer is a disease of these cells. Although cells in different parts of the body may look and work differently, most repair and reproduce themselves in the same way. Normally, this division of cells takes place in an orderly and controlled manner. If, for some reason, the process gets out of control, the cells will continue to divide, developing into a lump which is called a **tumour.** Tumours can be either **benign** or **malignant**.

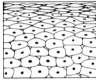
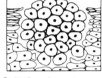

Normal cells   Cells forming a tumour

In a benign tumour the cells do not spread to other parts of the body and so are not cancerous. If they continue to grow at the original site, however, they may cause a problem by pressing on the surrounding organs.

A malignant tumour consists of cancer cells which have the ability to spread beyond the original site. If the tumour is left untreated, it may invade and destroy surrounding tissue. Sometimes cells break away from the original **(primary)** cancer and spread to other organs in the body through the bloodstream or lymphatic system. When these cells reach a new site they may go on dividing and form a new tumour, often referred to as a **secondary** or a **metastasis**.

Sometimes a cancer in the lung is a secondary from a cancer elsewhere in the body. In that case the treatment will depend on where the cancer first started. Your doctor will be able to tell you whether your cancer started in the lung (primary) or is a secondary tumour. This booklet deals only with primary lung cancer. If you have a cancer which has spread to the lung but started elsewhere in the body, then BACUP can send you a booklet about that particular cancer.

What are the symptoms of lung cancer?

The symptoms of lung cancer may include any of the following:

- A persistent cough or change in the nature of a long-standing cough
- A chest infection that does not get better
- Shortness of breath
- Coughing up blood-stained phlegm (sputum)
- Chest discomfort – this may be noticed as a dull ache or a sharp pain when you cough or take a deep breath
- Loss of appetite and loss of weight

If you do have any of the above symptoms, you must have them checked by your doctor. But remember, all of them occur in many conditions other than cancer.

What are the different types of lung cancer?

There are four common types of lung cancer. These are identified by looking at the cells of the cancer under a microscope.

- **Squamous cell carcinoma** is the commonest type of lung cancer. It comes from the cells which line the airways.
- **Adenocarcinoma** develops from the cells which produce mucus. These cells are also found in the lining of the airways.
- **Large cell carcinoma** gets its name from the large, rounded cells that are seen when they are examined under the microscope.

  The three types of lung cancer described above are classified under the name **'non-small cell lung cancer'** because their behaviour and response to treatment differs from the fourth type, which is:
- **Small cell** or **'oat cell' carcinoma**. It is called this because of its distinctive oat-shaped cells.

Another, less common, type of cancer which can affect the lungs is called **mesothelioma.** It is a cancer of the cells which line the lungs, known as the pleura, and is often linked to exposure to asbestos. This type of cancer is not discussed in this booklet, but BACUP has a factsheet about mesothelioma which we would be happy to send to you.

This booklet is about **primary lung cancer,** where the cancer has started in the lung. It should not be confused with **secondary lung cancer,** where cancer which started in another part of the body has spread to the lung. If you have secondary cancer of the lung, this booklet is not appropriate for you. Contact BACUP's information service if you would like to find out about secondary cancer of the lung.

How does the doctor make the diagnosis?

Most people begin by seeing their family doctor (general practitioner) who will examine you and arrange for you to have any further tests or X-rays. Your GP may need to refer you to the hospital for these tests and for specialist advice and treatment.

At the hospital the doctor will take your medical history before doing a physical examination. A chest X-ray will be taken to check for any abnormalities in your lungs. You may also be asked to bring samples of phlegm to the hospital so it can be examined under a microscope for cancer cells (sputum cytology).

The following tests are all used to diagnose cancer of the lung and your doctor may arrange for you to have one or more of them at the hospital.

Bronchoscopy

In this test the doctor examines the inside of the lung airways and takes cell samples (called **biopsies**). Normally, a thin, flexible tube called a **bronchoscope** is used, and the test is carried out under local anaesthetic. Sometimes a rigid bronchoscope is used instead. If this happens, a general anaesthetic is given, and you may have to stay in hospital overnight.

Before your bronchoscopy you will be asked not to eat or drink anything for a few hours. Just before the test you may be given a mild sedative, to help you relax and relieve any discomfort, and another medicine which reduces secretion. This medicine can make your mouth feel rather dry. Once you are comfortable a local anaesthetic will be sprayed onto the back of your throat. The **bronchoscope** is then gently passed through your nose or mouth and into the lung airways. The doctor can look through the bronchoscope to check for any abnormalities. Photographs and cell samples can be taken at the same time.

The test may be slightly uncomfortable but it only takes a few minutes. You shouldn't eat or drink for at least an hour afterwards because your throat will be numb and you wouldn't know if food and drink went down the wrong way. As soon as the sedation has worn off you will be able to go home. You should not drive for 24 hours after the test and should arrange for someone to collect you from hospital, as you may feel sleepy and have difficulty getting home. You may have a sore throat for a couple of days after your test but this will soon disappear.

Mediastinoscopy

This test allows the doctor to examine the area at the centre of the chest and local lymph nodes. The test is done under a general anaesthetic and will mean a short stay in hospital.

A small cut is made through the skin at the base of the neck and a tube, like a small telescope, is passed into the chest. The doctor can use this tube to examine the area. He or she may also take samples of the cells and lymph nodes for examination under a microscope.

Lung biopsy

This test is usually done in the X-ray department, most commonly during a CT scan (see page 13). A local anaesthetic is used to numb the area. Then you will be asked to hold your breath while a thin needle is passed through the skin into the lung. An X-ray is used to make sure that the needle is in the right position. A sample of cells is then taken for examination under a microscope.

The biopsy is sometimes slightly uncomfortable but it only takes a few minutes.

Further tests

If the tests show that you have cancer of the lung, your doctor may want to do some of the further tests described below to see if the disease has spread to other parts of your body. The results help your doctor to decide which is the best type of treatment for you.

CT scan (CAT scan)

In this scan several small X-rays are taken of the area in question and fed into a computer. This builds up a detailed picture of the size and position of the cancer.

Before the scan you will be asked to drink a special liquid which shows up on X-ray and ensures that a clear picture is obtained. Once you are lying in a comfortable position, the scan will be taken. The scan itself is painless but it will mean lying still for about 30-40 minutes.

You will probably be able to go home as soon as the scan is over.

Liver and upper abdominal ultrasound scan

This test is used to make up a picture of the liver and the other organs in the upper abdomen.

Before your test you will be asked to drink plenty of fluids so that your bladder is full and a clearer picture can be seen. Once you are lying comfortably on your back a gel is spread onto your abdomen. A small device, like a microphone, which produces sound waves, is then passed over the area. The sound waves are then converted into a picture by a computer.

This is a painless test and only takes a few minutes.

Isotope bone scan

Bone scans are very sensitive and can detect cancer cells before they show up on X-ray.

For this test a very small amount of a mildly radioactive substance is injected into a vein, usually in your arm. A scan is then taken of the affected area. As abnormal bone absorbs more of the radioactive substance than normal bone, this shows up on the scan as highlighted areas.

After the injection you will have to wait for up to three hours before the scan can be taken, so you may want to take a magazine or book with you, or a friend to keep you company.

The level of radioactivity used in these scans is very low and is not harmful. The radioactivity disappears from the body within a few hours.

Lung function tests

If your doctor wants to remove your lung cancer using surgery, s/he will first give you breathing tests to see how well your lungs are working.

It will probably take several days for the results of your tests to be ready and a follow-up appointment will be arranged for you before you go home. Obviously this waiting period will be an anxious time for you and it may help to talk things over with a close friend or relative. You may want to ring BACUP's cancer information service (phone numbers on pages 36 and 37) to ask any questions you may have.

What types of treatment are used?

Surgery, radiotherapy and chemotherapy may be used alone, or together, to treat cancer of the lung. Your doctor will plan your treatment by taking into consideration a number of factors including your general health, the type and size of the tumour, what it looks like under the microscope and whether it has spread beyond the lung.

You may find that other people at the hospital are having different treatment from yourself. This may be because their illness takes a different form and they have different needs. If you have any questions about your own treatment, don't be afraid to ask your doctor or the nurse looking after you. It often helps to make a list of questions for your doctor and to take a close friend or relative with you. You may want to use the fill-in page at the back of this booklet to write down your questions, and the answers you receive.

Some people find it reassuring to have another medical opinion to help them decide about their treatment. Most doctors will be pleased to refer you to another specialist for a second opinion if you feel this will be helpful.

Surgery

If the non-small cell lung cancer is small and has not spread, it may be possible to remove it with surgery.

The type of operation chosen will depend upon the size and position of the tumour.

- removal of a lobe of the lung is called a **lobectomy**
- removal of an entire lung is called a **pneumonectomy**

Occasionally, in patients whose lungs are not working well, a very small amount of the lung is removed. This is called a **wedge resection.** This operation is not done very often.

In small cell lung cancer, surgery is very rarely used, as the cancer has usually spread to other parts of the body before being diagnosed, even if it cannot be seen on the scan. Chemotherapy and/or radiotherapy are usually more effective.

People are often worried that they will not be able to breathe properly if their lung has been removed. **This is not so.** It is quite possible to breathe normally with only one lung, but people who had breathing difficulties before the operation may be more breathless afterwards. Breathing tests, which measure how well your lungs work, will be done to help you and your doctor decide whether an operation is right for you.

Before any operation, make sure that you have discussed it fully with your doctor so that you understand what it involves. Remember, no operation or procedure will be done without your consent.

Surgery may sometimes be combined with radiotherapy or chemotherapy. Details of these treatments are given on pages 17-22. BACUP will also be happy to send you publications specifically about them.

After your operation

It can take many weeks to recover fully from a lung operation, although some people recover more quickly than others. There are things you can do to help speed up your recovery. After your operation you will be encouraged to start moving about as soon as possible. This is an essential part of your recovery and even if you have to stay in bed it is important to keep up regular leg movements. A physiotherapist will visit you on the ward regularly to help you with breathing exercises.

A drip (intravenous infusion) will be used to replace your body fluids for a couple of days, until you are able to eat and drink again.

Drainage tubes will also be in place from your wound. These are usually removed about two to seven days after your operation. X-rays will be taken regularly to make sure your lung is working properly.

It is quite normal to have some discomfort after your operation. This can usually be controlled by giving pain-killing drugs. Let your doctor or one of the nurses know if you have any pain so they can treat it as soon as possible. Mild discomfort or pain in your chest can last for several weeks and you will be given some pain-killing tablets to take home with you.

You will probably be ready to go home about five to ten days after your operation. If you think you might have problems when you go home, for example if you live alone or have several flights of stairs to climb, let one of the nurses or the hospital social worker know when you are admitted to the ward, so that help can be arranged.

As well as being able to offer practical advice, many social workers are also trained counsellors and they can offer valuable support to you and your relatives, both in hospital and at home.

When you go home, it is important to exercise, to build up your strength and fitness. It is a good idea to check with your doctor or physiotherapist which kind of exercise would be suitable for you. Here are some exercise suggestions:

- brisk walks
- swimming
- jogging

Talk to your doctor or physiotherapist if you would like more information, or call BACUP's cancer information service (phone numbers on pages 36 and 37).

Before you leave hospital you will be given an appointment to attend an out-patient clinic for your post-operative check-up. This is a good time to discuss with your doctor any problems you may have after your operation.

If you have any worries or symptoms before your check-up, contact your doctor or the ward for advice.

Radiotherapy

Radiotherapy treats cancer by using high energy rays which destroy the cancer cells, while doing as little harm as possible to normal cells.

In non-small cell lung cancer, radiotherapy may be used as the main treatment, particularly where the cancer cannot be removed with an operation but has not spread. Radiotherapy may also be very effective in relieving symptoms, such as pain.

In small cell lung cancer, when the cancer has not spread outside the chest, giving radiotherapy after chemotherapy may improve the results. Radiotherapy may also be used very effectively to relieve symptoms, such as pain.

Sometimes, if people with small cell lung cancer have responded very well to chemotherapy, radiotherapy is given to the head to reduce the risk of the cancer spreading there.

Radiotherapy is usually given by directing rays from outside the chest onto the lung. Sometimes it is helpful to give a special form of radiotherapy called **endobronchial radiotherapy** or **brachytherapy.** This form of radiotherapy is given when the tumour is blocking one of the airways, causing the lung to collapse. It is a simple way of opening up the airway. If you have this type of radiotherapy, you usually need only one session of treatment.

Radiotherapy is given in the hospital radiotherapy department. The number of treatments you receive, and the length of time they take, will depend upon the type and size of the cancer.

External radiotherapy

To ensure that you receive maximum benefit from your radiotherapy, it has to be carefully planned. On your first few visits to the radiotherapy department you will be asked to lie under a large machine called a simulator, which takes X-rays of the area to be treated. Sometimes a CT scanner (see page 13) can be used for the same purpose. Treatment planning is a very important part of radiotherapy and it may take a few visits before the radiotherapist (the doctor who plans and supervises your treatment) is satisfied with the result.

Marks may be drawn on your skin to help the radiographer, who gives you your treatment, to position you accurately and to show where the rays are to be directed. These marks must remain visible throughout your treatment but they can be washed off once your course is over. At the beginning of your radiotherapy you will be given instructions on how to look after the skin around the area to be treated.

Before each session of radiotherapy the radiographer will position you carefully on the couch, either sitting or lying, and make sure you are comfortable. During your treatment, which only takes a few minutes, you will be left alone in the room but you will be able to talk to the radiographer who will be watching you carefully from an adjoining room. Radiotherapy is not painful but you do have to be still for a few minutes while your treatment is being given.

Internal radiotherapy

If you are having endobronchial radiotherapy, a thin tube (**catheter**) will be placed temporarily inside your lung using a bronchoscope (see page 11). The source of radiation will then be put inside the catheter.

Side effects

Radiotherapy can cause general side effects such as nausea, vomiting, diarrhoea and tiredness. It can also cause flu-like symptoms for a few days or chest pain. These side effects can be mild or more troublesome, depending on the strength of the radiotherapy dose and the length of your treatment. The radiotherapist will be able to advise you what to expect.

Nausea can usually be effectively treated by anti-sickness drugs (called anti-emetics), which your doctor can prescribe. If you don't feel like eating, you can replace meals with nutritious, high-calorie drinks which are available from most chemists and can be prescribed by your GP. BACUP's booklet *Diet and the cancer patient* has some helpful hints on how to eat well when you are feeling ill.

The main problem you are likely to notice, towards the end of your course of treatment, is that you have difficulty in swallowing. You may also find that drinking very hot or cold liquids is uncomfortable.

As radiotherapy can make you feel tired, try and get as much rest as you can, especially if you have to travel a long way for treatment each day.

All these side effects should disappear gradually once your course of treatment is over, but it is important to let your doctor know if they continue.

External radiotherapy does not make you radioactive and it is perfectly safe for you to be with other people, including children, throughout your treatment. Internal radiotherapy does make you slightly radioactive for a few days. This means that you will need to take certain safety measures. The hospital staff looking after you will explain these in more detail.

BACUP publishes a booklet called *Understanding radiotherapy*, which gives more details about this treatment and its side effects.

Chemotherapy

Chemotherapy is the use of special anti-cancer (cytotoxic) drugs to destroy cancer cells. They work by disrupting the growth of cancer cells.

In non-small cell lung cancer, chemotherapy may shrink the cancer in some people. The aims are to control symptoms and prolong good quality life.

Recently, in non-small cell lung cancer, chemotherapy has been used before surgery and radiotherapy to try and improve results. This is called neo-adjuvant chemotherapy. Clinical trials are now going on to find out how best to use this combination of treatments.

Chemotherapy is the main treatment for small cell lung cancer. In many cases small cell lung cancer will respond well to chemotherapy and it can be useful in improving quality of life and symptoms.

Chemotherapy may be given on its own, or before radiotherapy, to treat small cell lung cancers.

The drugs are sometimes given as tablets or, more usually, by injection into a vein **(intravenously)**. A course of chemotherapy usually lasts a few days. This is followed by a rest period of a few weeks, which allows your body to recover from any side effects of the treatment. The number of courses you have will depend on the type of cancer you have and how well it is responding to the drugs.

Chemotherapy may be given to you as an out-patient, but often it will mean spending a few days in hospital.

Side effects

Recent developments in the control of potential side effects of chemotherapy have made it much more tolerable than in previous years. Your doctor will tell you what problems, if any, to expect from your treatment.

While the drugs are acting on the cancer cells in your body they also reduce temporarily the number of normal cells in your blood. When these cells are in short supply you are more likely to get an infection and to tire easily. During chemotherapy your blood will be tested regularly and, if necessary, you will be given blood transfusions or antibiotics to treat any infection.

Some of the drugs used to treat lung cancer may cause nausea and vomiting. There are now very effective anti-sickness drugs (anti-emetics) to prevent or substantially reduce nausea and vomiting. Your doctor will prescribe these for you. Some chemotherapy drugs can make your mouth sore and cause small ulcers. Regular mouthwashes are important and the nurse will show you how to do these properly. If you don't feel like eating during treatment, you could try replacing some meals with nutritious drinks or a soft diet - BACUP's booklet *Diet and the cancer patient* has some useful tips on coping with eating problems.

Unfortunately, hair loss is another common side effect of some - but not all - of these drugs. Ask your doctor if the drugs you are taking are likely to cause hair loss or other specific side effects. People who lose their hair often cover up by wearing wigs, hats or scarves. Most patients are entitled to a free wig from the National Health Service and your doctor or nurse will be able to arrange for a wig specialist to visit you. If you do lose your hair, it will grow back surprisingly quickly.

BACUP has a booklet called *Coping with hair loss*, which you may find helpful

---

Although they may be hard to bear at the time, these side effects will disappear once your treatment is over.

Chemotherapy affects people in different ways. Some find they are able to lead a fairly normal life during their treatment, but many find they become very tired and have to take things much more slowly. Just do as much as you feel like and try not to overdo it.

BACUP's booklet *Understanding chemotherapy* discusses the treatment and its side effects in more detail. We would be pleased to send you a copy. Factsheets about individual drugs and their particular side effects are also available.

Laser therapy and airway stents

Sometimes lung cancer causes breathlessness by obstructing the wind pipe (the **trachea**) or one of the main airways which lead air from the wind pipe into the lungs. If the obstruction is caused by a tumour within the airway it can often be relieved by **laser therapy,** which burns the tumour out of the airway. Laser therapy does not destroy the tumour completely, but it does provide relief of symptoms.

Laser therapy is usually carried out under a general anaesthetic. While you are asleep a bronchoscopy (see page 11) is carried out and a flexible fibre is passed through the bronchoscope to aim the laser beam at the tumour. The laser beam is turned on and as much of the tumour as possible is burned away. The bronchoscope is then removed and you are brought round from the anaesthetic. Usually the anaesthetic is given into a vein and recovery from it is very rapid.

There are not usually any side effects from laser therapy. If the treatment has been straightforward you may be able to go home the same evening, or more often the next day. If there has been infection in your lung beyond the blockage that has been relieved by the laser treatment, it may be necessary for you to stay in hospital for a few days for antibiotics and physiotherapy.

If the obstruction to the airway recurs, the laser treatment can be repeated. Sometimes radiotherapy is given to try to prolong the relief provided by the laser therapy.

On other occasions an airway can become blocked by pressure on it from the outside, causing it to close. This can sometimes be relieved using a small device called a **stent**, which is placed inside the airway to hold it open. The most commonly used stent is a little wire frame, rather like a tiny umbrella. It is inserted through a bronchoscope in a folded up position and as it comes out of the end of the bronchoscope it opens up, pushing the walls of the narrowed airway open.

Stents are usually inserted under a general anaesthetic. When you wake up you will probably not notice that it is present, but you will be able to breathe more easily. The stent remains in your lung permanently and does not cause any problems.

Relief of symptoms

Apart from the symptoms which led you to consult your doctor in the first place, sometimes new symptoms, such as shortness of breath, can develop during your illness. These may be caused by the spread of the lung cancer to other parts of the body, but they may have another cause. For example, some lung cancer cells produce hormones which can upset the body's chemical balance. If you have any new symptoms, tell your doctor straight away so that you can be given treatment for them, or perhaps reassurance that they are nothing to worry about.

BACUP has a booklet called *Feeling better - controlling pain and other symptoms of cancer*, which you may also find helpful.

Follow up

After your treatment is completed your doctor will probably want you to have regular check-ups and X-rays. These often continue for several years. If you have any problems, or notice any new symptoms in between these times, let your doctor know as soon as possible.

New treatments

New ways to treat cancer of the lung are currently being studied.

New ways of giving radiotherapy, such as giving several doses a day, are being investigated in cases of non-small cell lung cancer. Also in non-small cell lung cancer, giving chemotherapy before surgery to improve the ability of the surgeon to completely remove the tumour is being investigated. Other studies are looking at giving chemotherapy before and during radiotherapy as well as after. Laser therapy for relieving blocked windpipes is being increasingly used.

Research – clinical trials

Research into new ways of treating cancer of the lung is going on all the time. As no current cancer treatment results in the cure of all the patients treated, cancer doctors are continually looking for new ways to treat the disease and they do this by using clinical trials. Many hospitals now take part in these trials. BACUP holds a list of some current trials and can put you in touch with the appropriate organisation or doctor.

If early work suggests that a new treatment might be better than the standard treatment, cancer doctors will carry out trials to compare the new treatment with the best available standard ones. This is called a controlled clinical trial and is the only reliable way of testing a new treatment. Often several hospitals around the country take part in these trials.

So that the treatments can be compared accurately, the type of treatment a patient receives is decided at random – typically, by a computer – and not by the doctor treating the patient. This is because it has been shown that if a doctor chooses the treatment, or offers a choice to the patient, he or she may unintentionally bias the result of the trial.

In a randomised controlled clinical trial, some patients will receive the best standard treatment while others will receive the new treatment, which may or may not prove to be better than the standard treatment. A treatment is better either because it is more effective against the tumour or because it is equally effective and has fewer unpleasant side effects.

The reason why your doctor would like you to take part in a trial (or study as they are sometimes called) is because until the new treatment has been tested scientifically in this way it is impossible for doctors to know which is the best one to choose for their patients.

Before any trial is allowed to take place it must have been approved by an ethics committee. Your doctor must have your informed consent before entering you into any clinical trial. Informed consent means that you know what the trial is about, you understand why it is being conducted and why you have been invited to take part, and you appreciate exactly how you will be involved.

**Even after agreeing to take part in a trial,
you can still withdraw at any stage
if you change your mind**

Your decision will in no way affect your doctor's attitude towards you. If you choose not to take part or you withdraw from a trial, you will then receive the best standard treatment rather than the new one with which it is being compared.

If you do choose to take part in a trial, it is important to remember that whatever treatment you receive will have been carefully researched in preliminary studies, before it is fully tested in any randomised controlled clinical trial. By taking part in a trial you will also be helping to advance medical science and so improve prospects for patients in the future.

BACUP has a booklet called *Understanding clinical trials,* which explains clinical trials in more detail. We would be happy to send you a copy.

Your feelings

Most people feel overwhelmed when they are told they have cancer. Many different emotions arise which can cause confusion and frequent changes of mood. You might not experience all the feelings discussed below or experience them in the same order. This does not mean, however, that you are not coping with your illness.

Reactions differ from one person to another – there is no right or wrong way to feel

---

These emotions are part of the process that many people go through in trying to come to terms with their illness. Partners, family members and friends often experience similar feelings and frequently need as much support and guidance in coping with their feelings as you do.

Shock and disbelief

'I can't believe it'; 'It can't be true'

This is often the immediate reaction when cancer is diagnosed. You may feel numb, unable to believe what is happening or to express any emotion. You may find that you can take in only a small amount of information and so you have to keep asking the same questions over and over again, or you need to be told the same bits of information repeatedly. This need for repetition is a common reaction to shock. Some people may find their feelings of disbelief make it difficult for them to talk about their illness with their family and friends. Others may feel an overwhelming urge to discuss it with those around them. This may be a way of helping them to accept the news themselves.

BACUP has a booklet called *Who can ever understand? – talking about your cancer,* which we would be happy to send to you.

Fear and uncertainty

'Am I going to die?'; 'Will I be in pain?'

Cancer is a frightening word surrounded by fears and myths. One of the greatest fears expressed by almost all newly diagnosed cancer patients is: 'Am I going to die?'

In fact, nowadays many cancers are curable if caught at an early enough stage. When a cancer is not completely curable, modern treatments often mean that the disease can be controlled for years and many patients can live an almost normal life.

Many people feel they need to sort out their affairs when they have been diagnosed with cancer, or any other potentially life-threatening illness. Doing so can take away some of that uncertainty, and reassure them that whatever happens their family will be looked after. One way to do this is to make a will, and BACUP has a booklet, *Will power,* which can help.

'Will I be in pain?' and 'Will any pain be unbearable?' are other common fears. In fact, many people with cancer feel no pain at all. For those who do, there are many modern drugs and other techniques which are very successful at relieving pain or keeping it under control. Other ways of easing pain or preventing you from feeling pain are radiotherapy and nerve blocks. BACUP's booklet *Feeling better – controlling pain and other symptoms of cancer* may help you understand more about these procedures. We will be happy to send this to you.

Many people are anxious about their treatment – whether or not it will work and how to cope with possible side effects. It is best to discuss your individual treatment in detail with your doctor. Make a list of questions you may want to ask (see fill-in form at the end of this booklet).

> ### If you don't understand something about your treatment - ask

You may like to take a close friend or relative to the appointment with you. If you are feeling upset, they may be able to remember details of the consultation which you might have forgotten. You may want them to ask some of the questions you yourself might be hesitant of putting to the doctor.

Some people are afraid of the hospital itself. It can be a frightening place, especially if you have never been in one before, but talk about your fears to your doctor; he or she should be able to reassure you.

You may find the doctors can't answer your questions fully, or that their answers may sound vague. It is often impossible to say for certain that they have completely removed the tumour. Doctors know from past experience approximately how many people will benefit from a certain treatment, but it is impossible to predict the future for a particular person. Many people find this uncertainty hard to live with – not knowing whether or not you are cured can be disturbing.

Uncertainty about the future can cause a lot of tension, but fears are often worse than the reality. Gaining some knowledge about your illness can be reassuring. Discussing what you have found out with your family and friends can help to relieve tension caused by unnecessary worry.

Denial

'There's nothing really wrong with me'; 'I haven't got cancer'

Many people cope with their illness by not wanting to know anything about it, or not wanting to talk about it. If that's the way you feel, then just say quite firmly to the people around you that you would prefer not to talk about your illness, at least for the time being.

Sometimes, however, it is the other way round. You may find that it is your family and friends who are denying your illness. They appear to ignore the fact that you have cancer, perhaps by playing down your anxieties and symptoms or deliberately changing the subject. If this upsets or hurts you because you want them to support you by sharing what you feel, try telling them. Start perhaps by reassuring them that you do know what is happening and that it will help you if you can talk to them about your illness.

Anger

'Why me of all people?'; 'And why right now?'

Anger can hide other feelings such as fear or sadness and you may vent your anger on those who are closest to you and on the doctors and nurses who are caring for you. If you have a religious faith you may feel angry with your God.

It is understandable that you may be deeply upset by many aspects of your illness and there's no need to feel guilty about your angry thoughts or irritable moods. However, relatives and friends may not always realise that your anger is really directed at your illness and not against them. If you can, it may be helpful to tell them this at a time when you are not feeling quite so angry, or if you would find that difficult, perhaps you could show them this section of the booklet. If you are finding it difficult to talk to your family, it may help to discuss the situation with a trained counsellor or psychologist. BACUP can give you details of how to get this sort of help in your area.

Blame and guilt

'If I hadn't ... this would never have happened'

Sometimes people blame themselves or other people for their illness, trying to find reasons why it should have happened to them. This may be because we often feel better if we know why something has happened, but since doctors rarely know exactly what has caused an individual's cancer, there's no reason for you to blame yourself.

Resentment

'It's all right for you, you haven't got to put up with this'

Understandably, you may be feeling resentful and miserable because you have cancer while other people are well. Similar feelings of resentment may crop up from time to time during the course of your illness and treatment for a variety of reasons. Relatives too can sometimes resent the changes that the patient's illness makes to their lives.

> ## Don't bottle up your feelings

It is usually helpful to bring these feelings out into the open so that they can be aired and discussed. Bottling up resentment can make everyone feel angry and guilty.

Withdrawal and isolation

'Please leave me alone'

There may be times during your illness when you want to be left alone to sort out your thoughts and emotions. This can be hard for your family and friends who want to share this difficult time with you. It will make it easier for them to cope, however, if you reassure them that although you may not feel like discussing your illness at the moment, you will talk to them about it when you are ready.

Sometimes depression can stop you wanting to talk. It may be an idea to discuss this with your GP, who can prescribe a course of antidepressant drugs or refer you to a doctor or counsellor who specialises in the emotional problems of people with cancer.

Learning to cope

After any treatment for cancer it can take a long time to come to terms with your emotions. Not only do you have to cope with the knowledge that you have cancer but also the physical effects of the treatment.

Although the treatment for cancer can cause unpleasant side effects many people do manage to lead an almost normal life during their treatment. Obviously you will need to take time off for it and some time afterwards to recover. Just do as much as you feel like and try to get plenty of rest.

Everyone needs some support during difficult times

It is not a sign of failure to ask for help or to feel unable to cope on your own. Once other people understand how you are feeling they can be more supportive.

What to do if you are a friend or relative

Some families find it difficult to talk about cancer or share their feelings. It may seem best to pretend that everything is fine, and carry on as normal, perhaps because you don't want to worry the person with cancer or feel you are letting him or her down if you admit to being afraid. Unfortunately, denying strong emotions like this can make it even harder to talk, and lead to the person with cancer feeling very isolated.

Partners, relatives and friends can help by listening carefully to what and how much the person with cancer wants to say. Don't rush into talking about the illness. Often it is enough just to listen and let the person with cancer talk when she or he is ready.

BACUP has a booklet, *Lost for words,* written for relatives and friends of people with cancer. It looks at some of the difficulties people may have when talking about cancer, and suggests ways of overcoming them.

Talking to children

Deciding what to tell your children about your cancer is difficult. How much you tell them will depend upon their age and how grown up they are. Very young children are concerned with immediate events. They usually need only simple explanations of why their relative or friend has had to go into hospital or isn't his or her normal self.

Slightly older children may understand a story explanation in terms of good cells and bad cells. All children need to be repeatedly reassured that your illness is not their fault because, whether they show it or not, children often feel they may somehow be to blame and may feel guilty for a long time. Most children of about 10 years old and over can grasp fairly complicated explanations.

Adolescents may find it particularly difficult to cope with the situation because they feel they are being forced back into the family just as they were beginning to break free and gain their independence.

An open, honest approach is usually the best way for all children. Listen to their fears and be aware of any changes in their behaviour. This may be their way of expressing their feelings. It may be better to start by giving only small amounts of information and gradually building up a picture of your illness. Even very young children can sense when something is wrong, so don't keep them in the dark about what is going on. Their fears of what it might be are likely to be far worse than the reality.

BACUP has a booklet called *What do I tell the children? – a guide for a parent with cancer,* which we would be happy to send you

---

What you can do

Many people feel helpless when they are first told they have cancer. They think there is nothing they can do, other than hand themselves over to doctors and hospitals. This is not so. There are many things you and your family can do at this time.

Understanding your illness

If you and your family understand your illness and its treatment, you will be better prepared to cope with the situation. In this way you at least have some idea of what you are facing.

For information to be of value it must come from a reliable source to prevent it causing unnecessary fears. Personal medical information should come from your own doctor, who is familiar with your medical background. As mentioned earlier, it can be useful to make a list of questions before you go to see the doctor or nurse, or take a friend or relative with you to remind you of things you want to know but can forget so easily. Other sources of information are given at the end of this booklet, along with a fill-in form to note your questions before your visit.

Practical and positive tasks

At times you may not be able to do things you used to take for granted. But as you begin to feel better you can set yourself some simple goals and gradually build up your confidence. Take things slowly and one step at a time.

Many people talk about 'fighting their illness'. This can help some people, and you can do it by becoming involved in your illness. One easy way of doing this is by planning a healthy, well-balanced diet. Another way is to learn relaxation techniques which you can practise at home with audiotapes. BACUP has booklets called *Cancer and complementary therapies* and *Diet and the cancer patient,* which we would be happy to send to you.

Some people find that their experience of cancer has taught them to prioritise their time and use their energy more constructively than they did before their illness.

You may find it helpful to take some regular exercise. The type of exercise you take, and how strenuous, depends on what you are used to and how well you feel. Set yourself realistic aims and build up slowly.

If the idea of changing your diet or taking exercise does not appeal to you, then do not feel you have to do these things; just do whatever suits you. Some people may find pleasure in keeping to their normal routine as much as possible. Others prefer to take a holiday or spend more time on a hobby.

Who can help?

The most important thing to remember is that there are people available to help you and your family. Often it is easier to talk to someone who is not directly involved with your illness. You may find it helpful to talk to a counsellor, who is specially trained to listen.

BACUP's cancer counselling service offers counselling at its London and Glasgow based offices

The counselling service can tell you more about counselling and can let you know what services are available in your area (see page 36). Some people find great comfort in religion at this time and it may help for them to talk to a local minister, hospital chaplain or other religious leader.

There are several other people who can offer support in the community. District nurses work closely with GPs and make regular visits to some patients and their families at home. In many areas of the country there are also Macmillan and Marie Curie nurses, who are specially trained to look after people with cancer in their own homes. Let your GP know if you are having any problems so that proper home care can be arranged.

Some hospitals have their own emotional support services with specially trained staff and some of the nurses on the ward will have been given training in counselling as well as being able to give advice about practical problems.

The hospital social worker is also often able to help in many ways such as giving information about social services and other benefits you may be able to claim while you are ill. For example, you may be entitled to meals on wheels, a home help or hospital fares. The social worker may also be able to help arrange childcare during and after treatment and, if necessary, help with the cost of childminders.

But there are people who require more than advice and support. They may find that the impact of cancer leads to depression, feelings of helplessness and anxiety. Specialist help in coping with these emotions is available in some hospitals. Ask your hospital consultant or GP to refer you to a doctor or counsellor who is an expert in the special emotional problems of cancer patients and their relatives.

Sick pay and benefits

Incapacity Benefit has replaced Invalidity Benefit and Sickness Benefit. There are three rates of Incapacity Benefit: a short-term lower rate, a short-term higher rate, and a long-term rate.

If you are employed and unable to work, your employer can pay you Statutory Sick Pay (SSP) for a maximum of 28 weeks. If, after this period, you are still unable to work, you can claim the short-term higher rate of benefit from the Benefits Agency. After one year, if you are still unable to work, you can claim long-term Incapacity Benefit.

If you are self-employed, you are entitled to the same benefits as long as you have been paying the relevant Class 2 contributions.

People who are unemployed and unable to work will need to transfer from the Job Seekers Allowance to the short-term lower rate of Incapacity Benefit.

If you are ill and not at work, do remember to ask your family doctor for a medical certificate to cover the period of your illness. If you are in hospital, ask the doctor or nurse for a certificate, which you will need to claim benefit. You may also be required to take a medical test to assess whether or not you are eligible for benefit.

You may qualify for the Disability Living Allowance. Ask your family doctor for form DS1500.

The Benefits Agency has a form (IB202) which outlines all these benefits and others to which you may be entitled. You can get a copy from your local Citizens' Advice Bureau and Social Security office, who will also be able to advise you about the benefits you can claim. Their addresses and telephone numbers are in the phone book.

CancerLink
11-21 Northdown Street, London N1 9BN
Tel: 0171 833 2818
    0800 132905 (Freephone helpline)
    0800 590415 (Asian language helpline)

Offers support and information on all aspects of cancer in response to telephone and letter enquiries. Acts as a resource to cancer support and self-help groups throughout the UK, and produces a range of publications on issues about cancer.

Cancer Care Society
21 Zetland Road, Redland, Bristol BS6 7AH
Tel: 0117 942 7419

Provides counselling and emotional support where possible through a network of support groups around the country. Holiday accommodation is available, and in some areas hospital visiting and help with transport.

Macmillan Cancer Relief
Anchor House, 15-19 Britten Street, London SW3 3TZ
Tel: 0171 351 7811
(with regional offices throughout the country)

Provides specialist advice and support through Macmillan nurses and doctors, and financial grants for people with cancer and their families.

Marie Curie Cancer Care
28 Belgrave Square, London SW1X 8QG
Tel: 0171 235 3325

Runs eleven hospice centres for cancer patients throughout the UK, and a community nursing service which works in conjunction with the district nursing service to support cancer patients and their carers in their homes.

National Radiological Protection Board (NRPB)
Chilton, nr Didcot, Oxfordshire OX11 0RQ
Tel: 0800 614529

Will carry out checks of radon levels in homes, free to households in radon-affected areas.

Tak Tent Cancer Support – Scotland
Block C20, Western Court,
100 University Place, Glasgow G12 6SQ
Tel: 0141 211 1932 (helpline/information)

*Offers information, support, education and care for cancer
patients, families, friends and professionals. Network of support
groups throughout Scotland. 'Drop-in' Resource and Information
Centre at the above address.*

Tenovus Cancer Information Centre
PO Box 88, College Buildings, Courtenay Road, Splott, Cardiff
CF1 1SA
Tel: 0800 526527 (freephone helpline)
        01222 497700 (admin)

*Provides an information service in English and Welsh on all
aspects of cancer, and emotional support for cancer patients and
their families. Operates a mobile screening unit, drop-in centre,
support group and cancer helpline.*

The Ulster Cancer Foundation
40-42 Eglantine Avenue, Belfast BT9 6DX
Tel: 01232 663439 (helpline)
        01232 663281 (admin)

*Provides a cancer information helpline and resource centre, and
support groups for patients and relatives. Produces a range of
booklets.*

Books recommended by BACUP

Cancer: a positive approach
Hilary Thomas and Karol Sikora
Thorsons, 1995
ISBN 0-7225-3132-X £8.99

Information about all aspects of cancer and the treatments available. Also looks at the controversies in cancer, and includes checklists of questions to ask your doctor.

Cancer: the facts
Michael Whitehouse & Maurice Slevin
Oxford University Press, 1996
ISBN 0-1926-1695-1 £8.99

Information on diagnosis and treatment of different types of cancer. Also considers the emotional needs of cancer patients, living with advanced cancer, and the role of complementary medicine.

Cancer: what every patient needs to know
Jeffrey Tobias
Bloomsbury, 1995
ISBN 0-7475-1993-5 £6.99

Thorough and up-to-date coverage by a respected cancer doctor.

Cancer information at your fingertips: the comprehensive cancer reference book for the 1990s (2nd edn)
Val Speechley and Maxine Rosenfield
Class Publishing, 1996
ISBN 1-872362-56-7 £11.95

Questions and answers about cancer, its diagnosis, treatment, side effects, complementary therapies and life with cancer.

Challenging cancer: from chaos to control
Nira Kfir and Maurice Slevin
Tavistock/Routledge, 1991
ISBN 0-415-06344-2 £12.99

For people who have been diagnosed with cancer, their families and friends. Examines feelings and emotions with the help of a psychotherapist and a cancer doctor. Suggests ways people can regain control of their lives.

Lung cancer: the facts
Chris Williams
Oxford University Press, 1992
ISBN 0-1926-2250-1 £6.99

Straightforward account of lung cancer, including causes, symptoms, diagnosis and treatments. Useful illustrations and a glossary explaining technical terms.

What you really need to know about cancer: a comprehensive guide for patients and their families
Robert Buckman
Macmillan, 1996
ISBN 0-333-61866-1 £20

Chapters on all types of cancer. Very comprehensive coverage, including sections on conventional and complementary treatments, screening, living with cancer and attitudes to cancer.

BACUP booklets

Understanding cancer series:

Acute lymphoblastic leukaemia
Acute myeloblastic leukaemia
Bladder
Bone cancer – primary
Bone cancer – secondary
Brain tumours
Breast – primary
Breast – secondary
Cervical smears
Cervix
Chronic lymphocytic leukaemia
Chronic myeloid leukaemia
Colon and rectum
Hodgkin's disease
Kaposi's sarcoma
Kidney
Larynx
Liver

Lung
Lymphoedema
Malignant melanoma
Mouth and throat
Myeloma
Non-Hodgkin's lymphoma
Oesophagus
Ovary
Pancreas
Prostate
Skin
Soft tissue sarcomas
Stomach
Testes
Thyroid
Uterus
Vulva

Understanding treatment series:

Bone marrow and stem cell
   transplants
Breast reconstruction
Chemotherapy

Clinical trials
Radiotherapy
Tamoxifen factsheet

Living with cancer series:

Complementary therapies
   and cancer
Coping at home: caring for
someone with advanced cancer
Coping with hair loss
Diet and the cancer patient
Facing the challenge of
   advanced cancer
Feeling better: controlling pain
   and other symptoms of cancer
Lost for words: how to talk to
   someone with cancer

Sexuality and cancer
What do I tell the children?
   – a guide for a parent with
   cancer
What now? Adjusting to life after
   cancer
Who can ever understand?
   – talking about your cancer
Will power – a step-by-step
   guide to making or changing
   your will

Notes

Questions you might like to ask your doctor or surgeon

You can fill this in before you see the doctor or surgeon, and then use it to remind yourself of the questions you want to ask, and the answers you receive.

1. ....

Answer ....

....

2. ....

Answer ....

....

3. ....

Answer ....

....

4. ....

Answer ....

....

5. ....

Answer ....

....

6. ....

Answer ....

....